NOURISH YOUR KIDNEYS, NOURISH YOUR LIFE

A Down-to-Earth Cookbook for Thriving with Chronic Kidney Disease

By

DR. KAREN R. MILLIRON

Disclaimer,

Copyright © by DR. KAREN R. MILLIRON 2024.. All rights reserved.

TABLE OF CONTENTS

INTRODUCTION

As a **nephrologist** with over two decades of experience, I've seen personally how nutrition can have a significant influence on the lives of people with chronic kidney disease (CKD). However, it wasn't until my own brother was diagnosed with stage 3 CKD that I realized the emotional and practical obstacles that patients and their families endure.

I recall John calling me, his voice shaking as he explained his diagnosis. As a vigorous 45-year-old father of two, he was overwhelmed by the idea of food limitations and the threat of illness progression. It was at that point that I understood how important it was to have a resource that not only gave medically solid dietary advice but also hope and empowerment.

"Nourish Your Kidneys, Nourish Your Life" is the result of this personal experience and professional competence. This cookbook is more than just a compilation of renal-friendly recipes; it's a comprehensive guide to living well with chronic kidney disease. Through these pages, I hope to simplify the complexity of renal nutrition and give you the skills you need to take charge of your health without sacrificing your enjoyment of food.

As we worked together to modify John's diet, I noticed his energy returning, his lab readings improving, and, most significantly, the spark rekindling in his eyes. I'd like to share this development with you. Each dish and piece of advice in this book is written with the knowledge that food is more than simply sustenance; it is an essential component of our cultural and emotional well-being.

Whether you're a recently diagnosed **CKD warrior, a long-time CKD warrior**, or **a caregiver** looking to help a loved one, this cookbook provides a recipe for tasty, kidney-nourishing meals that celebrate life. **<u>By adopting these concepts, you are not only managing a disease; you are going on a path to better health and energy.</u>**

Allow this book to be your friend as you face the challenges and triumphs of life with CKD. Together, we'll look at ways to nourish your kidneys and, by extension, your life. Remember that every meal is an opportunity to improve your health and enjoy the richness of life.

<u>Welcome to the next step in your renal health journey. Let us begin this gastronomic adventure together.</u>

CHAPTER 1

Understanding Kidney Health and Nutrition.

1.1 Diet and Chronic Kidney Disease.

As a nephrologist, I can verify that food is extremely important in controlling chronic kidney disease (CKD). The kidneys, which are responsible for filtering waste and excess fluid from the circulation, become weakened in CKD, demanding careful dietary control to alleviate the strain on these crucial organs and halt disease development.

Numerous studies have shown that dietary changes can help control CKD. For example, landmark research published in the New England Journal of Medicine (Klahr et al., 1994) found that a low-protein diet dramatically reduced renal disease development in individuals with mild renal insufficiency.

The foundation of nutritional management in CKD relies upon many essential nutrients:

1. Protein: While protein is necessary for basic processes, excessive protein metabolism generates nitrogenous waste, which overworked kidneys struggle to clear. A meta-analysis published in the Journal of the American Society of Nephrology by Fouque and Laville (2009) discovered that limiting protein consumption to 0.6-0.8 g/kg/day can halt GFR deterioration in non-diabetic individuals with CKD.

2. Sodium: restricting sodium intake is critical for maintaining blood pressure and minimizing fluid retention. The DASH-salt trial (Sacks et al., 2001) found that reducing salt consumption to 1,500 mg/day dramatically decreased blood pressure, a major determinant in CKD development.

3. Potassium: As CKD progresses, potassium excretion declines, threatening hyperkalemia. Research in the Clinical Journal of the American Society of Nephrology (Kovesdy et al., 2015) discovered that both high and low serum potassium levels were related to higher mortality in CKD patients, emphasizing the significance of careful potassium control.

4. **Phosphorus:** Phosphate retention begins early in CKD, contributing to secondary hyperparathyroidism and mineral bone disease. According to a study published in Kidney International (Block et al., 2004), higher serum phosphorus levels are independently related to increased mortality risk in CKD.

5. **Calcium:** While calcium consumption is frequently regulated to avoid vascular calcification, new study proposes a more nuanced approach. Research in the American Journal of Kidney Diseases (Hill et al., 2013) discovered that moderate calcium consumption may benefit CKD patients who are not yet on dialysis.

Surprisingly, new research has revealed the potential advantages of plant-based diets in CKD treatment.

The gut microbiome has emerged as a new arena for CKD research. Studies have demonstrated that uremic toxins generated by gut bacteria contribute to the pathogenesis of CKD. According to a review in Nutrients (Vaziri et al., 2016), dietary therapies targeting the gut flora may be a novel strategy for CKD management.

It is critical to understand that dietary requirements in CKD are not one-size-fits-all. They must be specific to the individual's CKD stage, comorbidities, and nutritional state. Regular monitoring of blood electrolytes, renal function, and nutritional indicators is required to adapt dietary recommendations as the condition advances.

In my clinical experience, I've found that patients who follow proper dietary guidelines have a higher quality of life, better control of CKD-related comorbidities, and, in some situations, a slower pace of disease development.

Empowering patients with information on the consequences of their eating choices may be transformative. It's not only about limitation; it's about making smart choices that promote renal health while still allowing you to enjoy your meals. This strategy, when paired with regular medical care and appropriate pharmaceutical therapies, is the basis of comprehensive CKD therapy.

1.2 Key Nutrients: Embrace and Limit.

Understanding which nutrients to consume and which to avoid is critical in the management of chronic kidney disease (CKD).

Let's look at the important actors in your dietary playbook:

Nutrients to embrace

1. **Fiber**: Often ignored in renal diets, fiber is an unsung champion. It helps regulate blood sugar and cholesterol levels, which is very useful for CKD patients who have diabetes or heart disease. Aim for 25-30 grams per day from foods such as berries, apples, and oats.
2. **Omega-3 fatty acids:** These anti-inflammatory powerhouses can help lower cardiovascular risk, which is a significant worry in CKD. Cold-water fish, such as salmon and mackerel, are good sources; nevertheless, check your nutritionist for recommended quantities.
3. **Antioxidants**: Vitamins C and E, along with other antioxidants, fight oxidative stress, which can exacerbate kidney disease. Berries,

bell peppers, and certain permitted nuts can be excellent sources.

4. <u>**Low-sodium herbs and spices**</u>: Enjoy taste without the sodium content. Herbs such as basil and oregano, as well as spices like turmeric, not only improve flavor but may also have anti-inflammatory properties.

Nutrients to Limit:

1. <u>**Sodium:**</u> The renal diet's infamous adversary. Excess salt can elevate blood pressure and cause fluid retention. Aim for fewer than 2,300 mg per day, or as recommended by your healthcare provider. Remember that salt may be found in unexpected areas, including bread and canned veggies.

2. <u>**Potassium:**</u> Potassium, while necessary for cardiac function, can accumulate to hazardous amounts in severe CKD. Foods high in potassium, such as bananas, oranges, and potatoes, may need to be reduced or avoided, depending on your specific needs.

3. <u>**Phosphorus:**</u> This mineral, which is plentiful in dairy products, almonds, and cola beverages, can lead to bone disease and cardiovascular difficulties if consumed in

excess. Your phosphorus requirements will vary according to your CKD stage and test findings.

4. <u>Protein:</u> It's a delicate balance; too little can cause malnutrition, while too much might overwork your kidneys. Your doctor will assist you in determining your optimal protein intake, which normally ranges between 0.6 and 0.8 g/kg body weight per day for non-dialysis individuals.

5. <u>**Advanced Glycation End Products (AGEs):**</u> These hazardous substances, which occur when meals are cooked at high temperatures, can cause inflammation and oxidative stress. Instead of frying or grilling, choose milder cooking methods such as steaming or boiling.

Remember that your dietary demands are as unique as your fingerprints. What works for one individual with CKD may not be appropriate for another. Regular check-ins with your healthcare team can help you fine-tune your diet as your illness progresses.

By consuming nutrient-dense, kidney-friendly foods and being aware of potential dietary traps, you are actively engaging in your therapy. This proactive strategy can result in improved results and a higher quality of life as you progress through your CKD journey.

1.3 Understanding Nutrition Labels for Kidney Health.

When dealing with chronic kidney disease (CKD), navigating grocery store aisles can feel like a minefield. However, learning the art of reading nutrition labels will be your hidden weapon on the dietary battlefield. Let's clear up any confusion about this important ability that can have a big influence on your kidney health.

To begin, realize that the Nutrition Facts label provides information about the ingredients of packaged items. It's more than simply a tangle of data; it's a guide to making educated decisions.

Here's how to successfully decode it:

Serving Size: This is the starting point.Be aware that many products include several servings. If you eat the full packet, multiply the specified values appropriately.

Calories: While calories are rarely a significant concern in CKD therapy, keeping track of them can help you maintain a healthy weight, which is good for your kidneys overall.

Now, let's focus on the nutrients that are particularly important for renal patients:

<u>Sodium:</u> This is frequently the first thing CKD patients should examine. Aim for foods that contain less than 140 mg of salt per serving. Be aware of words like "reduced sodium"; these items may still include a high sodium content when compared to fresh, unprocessed alternatives.

<u>Potassium</u> isn't often indicated on labels, despite its role in CKD treatment. When it is stated, search for alternatives that have less than 200 mg per serving, unless your dietician advises otherwise.

<u>Phosphorus</u>: Like potassium, phosphorus is not typically listed on labels. When listed, try for fewer than 50 mg per serving. Be wary of phosphorus additions in ingredient lists, which are commonly identified by the prefix "phos-" (e.g., phosphoric acid, sodium phosphate).

<u>Protein</u> requirements vary according to your CKD stage and if you are on dialysis. In general, most meals should have a reasonable protein concentration of 5–10 g per dish.

<u>Fiber</u> is often disregarded, yet it might be good for renal sufferers. Choose foods with at least 3 g of fiber per serving to promote digestive health and help regulate blood sugar and cholesterol levels.

<u>Total Carbohydrates</u>: While carbohydrate consumption is not normally limited in CKD diets, it is significant for people who are diabetic and have renal disease. When feasible, opt for complex carbs and whole grains.

Ingredients:

This is your investigative tool. Ingredients are given in descending order of weight. Beware of hidden sugars, sodium-based preservatives, and phosphorus additions.

<u>Now, let's talk about strategy. When comparing the products:</u>

1. <u>Standardized serving sizes:</u> When comparing two items with varied serving sizes, match the figures to provide a fair comparison.
2. <u>Look past the front of the package</u>: Terms like "natural" or "healthy" are unregulated and may be deceptive. Always check the Nutrition Facts label.
3. <u>Be wary of nutrient claims</u>: "low sodium" implies 140 mg or less per serving; however, "reduced sodium" just means 25% less than

the usual version, which might still be excessive.

4. <u>Look for hidden phosphorus</u>: Phrases like "seasoned," "processed," or "restructured" frequently imply extra phosphorus.

5. <u>Consider fresh alternatives:</u> Many entire foods, such as fruits and vegetables, do not have labels yet are typically the greatest options for kidney health.

Developing label-reading abilities requires effort, but it is a worthwhile investment in your health. Over time, you will become more efficient and confident in your decisions. Do not hesitate to bring labels to your dietician sessions for specific advice.

<u>Remember,</u> reading labels isn't about discovering **"perfect" meals**; <u>it's about making educated decisions that support your renal health objectives.</u> It is OK to eat items that do not meet all of the criteria on occasion. The idea is to maintain an overall balance and consistency in your diet.

Mastering nutrition labels allows you to be an active participant in your renal health journey, rather than a passive consumer. This information enables you to make decisions that benefit your health, one food item at a time. So, next time you're in the grocery store, take a moment to read the labels. Your kidneys will appreciate you for it.

1.4 Meal Planning Strategies for Optimal Renal Function.

Effective meal planning is critical for CKD patients to maintain peak renal function and overall health.

Here are some important techniques based on clinical research and patient outcomes.

1. Balanced Macronutrient Distribution: Research shows that a well-balanced diet can delay CKD development. Aim for this:

50-60% of calories come from complex carbs.

20-30% from lean proteins (modified according to CKD stage).

20-30% of heart-healthy fats

2. Portion Control: Using the plate technique simplifies meal planning.

1/2 plate of non-starchy veggies.

1/4 plate of lean protein.

One-quarter plate of complex carbs

This strategy aids with calorie control and nutritional balance.

3. Meal Frequency: Studies show that eating 4-6 smaller meals throughout the day can help stabilize blood sugar levels, reduce kidney workload, and improve nutritional utilization.

4. Strategic Protein Timing: Evenly distributing protein consumption between meals helps improve nitrogen balance and minimize renal stress. This is especially important for people in later stages of CKD.

5. Mindful Sodium Management: Limit sodium intake to 2,000-3,000 mg per day (varies by individual). Strategies include using herbs and spices for seasoning, reading product labels, and preparing meals at home to reduce salt.

6. Track Potassium and Phosphorus: Use a points system to monitor consumption of these nutrients. This clinically verified strategy allows patients to better visualize their daily boundaries.

7. Fluid Management: Adjust fluid intake according to urine output and CKD stage. Aim for 4-6 cups (32-48 ounces) for individuals with regular urine production.

Stricter limitations for people with severe kidney disease or on dialysis.

8. **Meal Preparation Techniques:**

Use cooking methods that conserve nutrients and reduce toxic compounds:

Steam or boil veggies to lower potassium content. - Avoid high-temperature cooking for proteins to prevent AGE development.

9. **Coordinate with healthcare providers** to integrate required supplements into meal planning, such as vitamin D and iron.

B-complex vitamins.

10. Diabetic CKD patients should consume low-glycemic index meals to properly maintain blood sugar levels.

Patients who apply these evidence-based treatments can considerably improve their nutritional status while potentially slowing the course of CKD. It is critical to note that these tactics must be adapted to the specific needs of each patient and altered on a frequent basis depending on test findings and clinical state.

Successful meal planning requires a collaborative effort from patients, nutritionists, and the entire nephrology care team. Regular follow-ups and dietary counseling sessions are critical for maximizing results and ensuring compliance with these renal-protective methods.

CHAPTER 2

The Basics of Kidney-Friendly Cooking

2.1 Essential Ingredients for a Kidney-Friendly Kitchen.

I will discuss the key components for a kidney-friendly kitchen. This information is based on current medical standards as well as nephrology nutrition research.

2.1 Essential Ingredients for a Kidney-Friendly Kitchen.

Creating a kidney-friendly kitchen begins with storing the necessary items. These options are designed to promote kidney health while also offering nutritional balance and taste variation.

1. **<u>Protein sources:</u>**

Lean meats: chicken breast, turkey, and lean cuts of beef (in moderation).

Salmon, trout, and tuna (canned in water)

Plant-based: tofu, tempeh, and beans (in limited quantities)

Egg whites.

Rationale: These supply vital amino acids while reducing saturated fat and phosphorus levels. The National Kidney Foundation recommends 0.6-0.8 g protein per kg body weight for non-dialysis CKD patients.

2. **<u>Complex carbs:</u>**

Rice: white, wild, or brown (depending on potassium levels)

Pasta (enriched white or whole grain)

Bread: reduced sodium variations

Oatmeal with barley

Rationale: These give calories and fiber while containing less potassium than other grains. Fiber intake of 25–30 g/day is advised for CKD patients to improve gut health and blood sugar control.

3. Vegetables: Low potassium alternatives include bell peppers, onions, garlic, cucumbers, and lettuce.

Cruciferous vegetables: cabbage and cauliflower (in moderation).

Green beans and carrots (cooked to minimize potassium).

Rationale: These give important vitamins and antioxidants while regulating potassium consumption. The Journal of Renal Nutrition recommends twice boiling high-potassium vegetables to lower potassium levels by up to 50%.

4. **Fruits** include apples, berries, pineapple, and grapes.

canned fruits in water or juice (drained).

Rationale: These provide critical vitamins and fiber while being low in potassium. The American Journal of Kidney Diseases suggests that most CKD patients restrict their fruit intake to 2-3 servings per day.

5. <u>Healthy fats:</u>

Olive oil or canola oil

Avocado (in limited quantities).

Unsalted nuts and seeds (in moderation)

Rationale: These include heart-healthy lipids and aid in the absorption of fat-soluble vitamins. The National Kidney Foundation recommends that 30% of your calories come from healthy fats.

6. **<u>Dairy alternatives</u>** include unsweetened almond milk and rice milk.

Non Dairy creamers (no phosphate additions)

Rationale: Compared to dairy, they have more calcium and less phosphorus. Excess phosphorus consumption has been linked to increased mortality in CKD patients, according to research.

7. **<u>Herbs and Spices:</u>** Fresh herbs include basil, cilantro, parsley, and oregano.

Spices: turmeric, cinnamon, garlic, and onion powder

Rationale: These provide taste without including salt. According to research published in the Clinical Journal of the American Society of Nephrology, herbs and spices can help CKD patients lower their salt intake.

8. **Beverage options** include water, herbal teas, and unsweetened cranberry juice.

Rationale: Proper hydration is essential, although fluid intake may be restricted in advanced CKD. The American Society of Nephrology suggests tailoring fluid consumption based on urine output and CKD stage.

9. Specialty items:

Ingredients: low-sodium broth, vinegars (apple cider, balsamic), and lemon juice.

Rationale: They enhance taste without jeopardizing renal health. Research published in the Journal of Renal Nutrition discovered that taste enhancers can boost dietary compliance in CKD patients.

It is important to remember that individual requirements may differ depending on CKD stage, comorbidities, and laboratory results. Always get tailored counsel from a nephrologist or renal dietician. When adopting dietary adjustments, it is critical to evaluate blood electrolytes regularly, particularly potassium and phosphorus levels.

Patients who store these kidney-supportive goods may prepare delightful, healthy meals that correspond with their renal health objectives. **Remember that moderation and portion control are important elements in CKD dietary management.**

2.2 Cooking Techniques that Preserve Nutrients and Flavor.

Evidence-based cooking methods that conserve nutrients while adhering to renal dietary recommendations.

1. **Blanching and double boiling: For potassium-rich vegetables:**

Blanch in boiling water for 1 minute before transferring to ice water.

Double boiling can lower potassium levels by 50–70% in vegetables such as potatoes, carrots, and squash.

2. **Steaming benefits vegetables and fish** by preserving water-soluble vitamins better than boiling. Use a steamer basket to avoid direct contact with water.

Steaming maintains up to 90% of water-soluble vitamins, whereas boiling can result in losses of up to

50% (Slow cooking is ideal for tougher types of meat. Use low-sodium broths or water-based liquids.

Add herbs and spices for taste without salt.

3.**Nutritional benefit**: This process breaks down difficult proteins, making them simpler to digest especially for CKD patients who may have compromised digestive function.

4. **Grilling and Broiling:** Suitable for meat and vegetables.

   Prevents hazardous chemicals from forming by avoiding charring.

5. **Stir-frying:**

Cook quickly to retain nutrients. Use tiny amounts of heart-healthy oils like olive oil.

Perfect for combining proteins and low-potassium veggies.

6. **Herb Infusion:** Steep fresh herbs in olive oil or vinegar to increase taste without adding sodium. high in antioxidants, which are excellent for kidney health..

7. **Pressure Cooking**: Reduces cooking time and protects heat-sensitive nutrients.

Effective for decreasing phosphorus levels in beans and legumes.

8. **Microwaving: Quick** cooking helps keep nutrients; use microwave-safe containers.

Suitable for reheating without adding additional fats or liquids.

Contrary to common assumption, microwaving can maintain nutrients better than other traditional cooking techniques due to its shorter cooking time.

9. **Roasting:** Ideal for vegetables and lean meats; improves taste without adding sodium; use a rack to drain fat.

Roasting at lower temperatures (about 350°F/175°C) will help reduce the production of advanced glycation end products (AGEs), which are especially problematic in CKD patients.

10. **Poaching** is a gentle way for cooking fish and poultry that uses herbs and lemon for taste instead of salt. It also retains moisture in proteins without adding fat.

Clinical relevance: This approach is very useful for CKD patients who need to decrease their salt and saturated fat consumption.

Remember that, while these strategies aid in the preservation of nutrients and the management of essential electrolytes, cooking methods must be tailored to individual dietary demands. Always check with your healthcare team, including a renal dietitian, to confirm that these strategies are appropriate for your unique dietary needs and CKD treatment strategy.

Using these evidence-based cooking techniques, you can prepare kidney-friendly meals that are both healthy and enjoyable, promoting overall health while following renal dietary requirements.

2.3 Herb and Spice Blends to Enhance Low-Sodium Flavor.

I'm pleased to offer some innovative herb and spice mixes that can boost flavor without jeopardizing renal health. These mixes are based on expertise and research into flavor profiles that appeal to patients with impaired taste perception due to CKD.

1. Renal Zest Blend.

Ingredients: 2 tablespoons dried lemon zest, 1 tablespoon dried orange zest, and 1 teaspoon garlic powder.

One teaspoon onion powder

1/2 teaspoon white pepper.

This citrus-forward combination has a bright, tangy flavor that may help alleviate the metallic sensation that some CKD patients feel. The zest provides taste without the acidity of the juice, which is beneficial for those with acid-base imbalances.

2. Kidney-Friendly Herbs of Provence

Ingredients: 2 tablespoons dried thyme, 1 tablespoon dried basil, and 1 tablespoon dried oregano.

Ingredients: 1 teaspoon dried lavender buds, 1/2 teaspoon fennel seeds.

This Mediterranean-inspired combination is high in antioxidants. Thyme, in example, has been proven in animal studies to have possible renoprotective properties; nevertheless, additional study in humans is needed.

3. Nephrotic Spice Mixture:

Ingredients: 1 tablespoon turmeric, 1 teaspoon coriander, 1 teaspoon cumin, 1/2 teaspoon ginger, and 1/4 teaspoon cinnamon.

Turmeric, the headline ingredient in this combination, has anti-inflammatory qualities that may benefit CKD patients. However, because of its high oxalate level, it should be used in moderation.

4. Dialysis Friendly Taco Seasoning:

1 tablespoon chili powder (no added salt)

1 teaspoon paprika.

Ingredients: 1 tsp ground cumin, 1/2 tsp garlic powder.

1/2 teaspoon onion powder.

1/4 teaspoon dried oregano.

This combination has the flavor of classic taco seasoning but without the excessive salt level. It's especially beneficial for those who miss Mexican food owing to dietary constraints.

To make Renal Roast Rub, combine 2 tbsp dried rosemary, 1 tbsp dry thyme, 1 tsp garlic powder, and 1 tsp onion powder.

1/2 teaspoon ground black pepper.

This combination is ideal for roasted meats and vegetables, providing a savory taste profile without the additional phosphates common in conventional meat seasonings.

6. CKD-Friendly Curry Powder

One tablespoon of ground coriander

Ingredients: 1 tsp ground cumin and 1 tsp ground turmeric.

1/2 teaspoon ground cardamom.

1/4 teaspoon ground cinnamon.

1/8 teaspoon ground cloves.

This mild curry combination provides diverse tastes without the spice that might aggravate gastrointestinal difficulties in certain CKD patients. It's also lower in potassium than commercial curry powders.

7. Phosphate-free poultry seasoning:

Ingredients: 2 tbsp dried sage, 1 tbsp dry thyme, 1 tsp dried marjoram, 1/2 tsp dried rosemary, and 1/4 tsp grated nutmeg.

This mix does not contain the phosphate additions commonly found in commercial chicken spices, making it safer for patients who are watching their phosphorus consumption.

8. Renal-Friendly Italian Blend.

Add 1 tbsp dried basil, 1 tbsp dry oregano, 1 tsp dried thyme, 1 tsp dried rosemary, and 1/2 tsp garlic powder.

This flexible mix may be used in a variety of recipes, capturing the spirit of Italian food without adding salt or phosphates.

When utilizing these mixtures, keep in mind that individual tolerances might differ. Begin with little quantities and adjust to taste. It's also important to examine the cumulative impact of herbs and spices, particularly those with diuretic characteristics or high oxalate levels.

These innovative mixes not only improve flavor but also the whole eating experience for CKD patients. We can increase dietary adherence in chronic renal disease treatment by offering a variety of enticing taste alternatives.

2.4 Portion Control and Balanced Meal Composition.

Picture this: You're sitting down to dinner, and instead of worrying about what you can and cannot eat, you feel confident and strong. That is the strength of good portion management and balanced meal composition. It's not only about limitations; it's about liberation via knowledge.

The Plate Method: A Visual Guide for Success

Imagine your plate is a painting, and you are the artist. Here is how to paint a masterpiece.

Half plate: bright, low-potassium veggies (such as colorful bell peppers, crisp cucumbers, or soft green beans).

1/4 plate of lean protein (a chunk the size of your hand)

1/4 plate: Complex carbs (similar to a cupped handful).

This easy visual guide eliminates the guesswork from portioning, enabling you to enjoy your meal.

Mindful Eating: Connecting With Your Food

In my work, I've witnessed patients change their attitudes toward food via mindful eating. Here's how.

Take a minute to appreciate your meal. Chew carefully and relish each bite.This method not only promotes digestion, but it also makes you feel more satiated with adequate meals.

The Power of Protein: Quality vs. Quantity

Protein is a double-edged sword for people with chronic kidney disease. Too much can strain the kidneys, while too little might cause muscular wastage.

The key is balance.

Focus on high-quality proteins (lean meats, seafood, egg whites).

Spread protein consumption equally throughout the day. - A portion should be around the size of a deck of cards.

Remember that it is not about deprivation but about fueling your body to its full potential.

Carbohydrates: Fueling the Day

Carbohydrates frequently receive a poor name, although they are necessary for energy. Choose wisely.

Choose complex carbohydrates, such as whole grains, in moderation.

A portion of grains should be the size of a clenched fist.

Balancing Act: The Art of Combination.

Creating a balanced meal is like leading an orchestra; each component plays an important part.

Include protein, carbohydrates, and healthy fats in every meal.

Use a range of textures and colors to make food appetizing.

Remember to add kidney-friendly fruits for dessert.

Emotional Connection: Food as Medicine.

In my years of work, I've seen how the appropriate approach to eating can boost morale and create optimism. Sarah, one of my patients, told me, "**Learning to eat this way not only improved my lab results, but it also gave me back control of my life.**"

Remember that each food is a chance to nurture both your body and your spirit. By mastering portion management and balanced meal composition, you are not just controlling a condition but also embracing a lifestyle that promotes your general well-being.

As we continue on our road, keep in mind that perfection is not the aim; progress is. Be gentle with yourself, appreciate minor achievements, and keep in mind that each balanced meal is one step closer to a healthier, happier you.

In the next part, we will look at several intriguing recipes that put these concepts into effect. Are you prepared to go on this delectable adventure? Let's cook up a storm in a kidney-friendly manner!

CHAPTER 3

Comprehensive Recipe Collection.

3.1 Nutritional Breakfast Options

Rise and shine with nourishing morning delights!

A healthy breakfast is sometimes overlooked in today's fast-paced world. However, this essential breakfast sets the tone for the rest of the day, preparing your body and mind for the difficulties that lie ahead.

Let's look at a breakfast choice that is not only healthy but also tasty and filling.

Introducing the Powerhouse Breakfast Bowl:

Imagine a brilliant, colorful dish filled with a variety of nutritious foods. At its core is a big scoop of creamy Greek yogurt, a protein powerhouse that keeps hunger at bay until noon. The acidic taste profile of the yogurt makes it an ideal canvas for the diversity of toppings that will follow.

Imagine a handful of mixed berries scattered on top of the yogurt, including lush blueberries, juicy strawberries, and tart raspberries. These jewel-toned fruits not only offer a burst of natural sweetness, but they also contain a lot of antioxidants, which help your immune system and general wellness.

Next, add a sprinkle of homemade granola for a delightful crunch with each scoop. This granola, made with rolled oats, almonds, and a touch of honey, provides complex carbs and heart-healthy lipids for breakfast. These components provide slow-release energy, keeping you focused and alert throughout the morning.

To improve the nutritional profile even further, add a tablespoon of chia seeds. These small powerhouses are loaded with omega-3 fatty acids, fiber, and minerals. As they absorb fluids, they produce a nice texture while also aiding digestion and energy levels.

Finally, pour a teaspoon of pure maple syrup on top for a natural sweetness that balances the sharpness of the yogurt and berries. This modest indulgence makes the bowl feel more like a pleasure than a nutritious dish, making you look forward to your breakfast.

The appeal of this Powerhouse Breakfast Bowl is not just its nutritious worth but also its adaptability. Ingredients can be readily swapped depending on seasonal availability or personal tastes. Use different varieties of yogurt, experiment with different fruits, or add other superfoods like goji berries or cacao nibs.

By taking a few minutes to prepare this nutrient-dense breakfast, you're investing in your health and establishing a good tone for the day ahead. It's a simple yet effective method to fuel your body, satisfy your taste buds, and recognize the necessity of getting your day started well.

3.2 Delicious Lunch and Dinner Entrees

A Globally Appealing Entree: Mediterranean Vegetable and Chickpea Stew.

This substantial Mediterranean-inspired stew has a balanced combination of flavors and textures that will appeal to a wide range of cultural tastes.

Here's what makes it a generally acceptable lunch or supper option:

1. The stew is easily adaptable to different nutritional choices, making it suitable for vegetarians, vegans, and meat eaters alike.
2. **Nutrient-dense ingredients**: Packed with veggies and legumes, it has a healthy balance of proteins, complex carbs, and important vitamins and minerals.
3. **Mild yet tasty profile**: The blend of herbs and spices provides depth without overpowering heat, making it suitable for a wide variety of taste preferences.
4. **Cultural fusion**: Inspired by Mediterranean cuisine, which is a melting pot of tastes, this dish bridges culinary barriers across areas.
5. **Affordability**: By using readily available ingredients, it is a cost-effective solution for many homes throughout the world.
6. **Convenience:** Because this recipe only requires one pot to prepare, it is ideal for busy individuals or families.
7. **Seasonal adaptability:** The recipe may be changed to use locally available food, making it useful year-round in a variety of regions.

8. **Health benefits**: High in fiber, antioxidants, and plant-based proteins, it meets many modern dietary guidelines.

This stew is a warm, healthy, and versatile alternative that may be enjoyed by a variety of groups throughout the world. Do you like me to offer a full recipe or elaborate on any aspect of this entree?

3.3 Healthy Side Dishes and Salads.

Healthy Side Dishes and Salads: Enhancing Your Meal with Nutrient-Rich Companions

Side dishes and salads are essential for balanced eating since they provide nutritional support while also bringing colorful tastes and textures to your main entrée.

Let's look at several solutions that stand out for their health advantages and broad appeal:

1. **Roasted rainbow root vegetables**.

This vibrant blend of carrots, parsnips, and beets serves as a visual feast while also providing a strong balance of vitamins and minerals. The roasting method caramelizes natural sugars, increasing tastes while preserving nutritional value. A little drizzle of olive oil and a sprinkling of fresh herbs elevates this side dish to gourmet level.

2. Quinoa Tabbouleh.

This protein-packed take on a Middle Eastern favorite replaces traditional bulgur with quinoa, a complete protein source. It's a delicious salad packed with fresh parsley, mint, tomatoes, and cucumber that may also be served as a light lunch. The lemony dressing provides brightness, making it an ideal accompaniment to heavier main courses.

3. Kale and Brussels sprout slaw.

This crisp slaw, made from two nutritious powerhouses, is a welcome counterpoint to milder meals. Kale and Brussels sprouts are mixed with tangy yogurt sauce, toasted almonds, and dried cranberries. It's a celebration of textures and an excellent way to get extra leafy greens into your diet.

4. Lentil & Roasted Bell Pepper Salad

This robust salad combines protein-rich lentils and sweet, smoky roasted bell peppers. It's dressed with balsamic vinaigrette and topped with crumbled feta for a delicious combination of flavors and textures. The lentils give prolonged energy, making this a great option for individuals looking for something more satisfying.

5. Asian-inspired cucumber salad

This salad is light and delicious, with thinly sliced cucumbers marinated in sesame-ginger dressing. The inclusion of edamame beans increases the protein level, and toasted sesame seeds offer a nutty bite. It provides a refreshing contrast to spicy main courses and is an excellent way to remain hydrated.

These healthy sides and salads not only complement your main courses but also stand on their own. They provide a variety of nutrients, tastes, and textures that may elevate an average meal into a complete gastronomic experience. Incorporating these nutrient-dense alternatives does more than simply add color to your plate; it also invests in your general health and well-being.

The secret to a good and nutritious dinner is frequently found in the balance between your main course and these properly prepared side dishes. Do you want more information on any of these dishes or ideas for how to match them with certain entrees?

3.4 Kidney-Friendly Snacks and Appetizers

Nutritional Bites for Renal Health

Finding appropriate snacks and appetizers might be difficult for those who are maintaining their renal health.

Here's a list of kidney-friendly foods that are both tasty and appropriate for renal diets:

1. **Apple and unsalted almond slices**.

Apples are low in salt and potassium yet give a delightful crunch. This snack, served with a modest piece of unsalted almonds, provides healthy fats and fiber without overloading on phosphorus or potassium.

2. **Rice cakes with hummus**.

Choose low-sodium rice cakes and top with a thin layer of homemade or low-sodium hummus. This combination creates a light, crispy snack that is kind on the kidneys.

3. **Cucumber rounds with herb cream cheese.**

Cucumbers are low in potassium and pleasantly crisp. Top thin slices with a tiny bit of herb-infused cream cheese for a delightful snack that is good for your kidneys.

4. Egg White and Red Bell Pepper Bites.

Egg whites are a great low-phosphorus protein source. Mix them with finely chopped red bell peppcr, bakc in tiny muffin pans, and you'll have a protein-rich, kidney-friendly snack.

5. Air-popped popcorn without salt is an excellent low-potassium, low-phosphorus snack. Season with herbs like rosemary or thyme for a flavor boost without adding salt.

6. Berries with Mint Salad

Berries, particularly strawberries and blueberries, are lower in potassium than other fruits. Mix them with fresh mint for a pleasant, kidney-friendly dessert.

7. Cauliflower "wings"

Lightly breaded and baked cauliflower florets will fulfill your yearning for something crunchy. Serve with a dipping sauce that is low in salt and kidney-friendly.

8. Zucchini chips

Thinly sliced zucchini, gently seasoned and cooked until crisp, is an excellent alternative to potato chips that have less potassium and phosphorus.

9. Red grapes with low-fat string cheese.

This traditional combo strikes a decent mix of sweetness and protein while remaining careful of potassium and phosphorus levels.

10. Garlic Herb Pita Chips.

Homemade pita chips, seasoned with garlic and herbs instead of salt, give a pleasant crunch without the added sodium.

When cooking these snacks, keep portion proportions in mind as well as specific dietary limitations. Always contact a renal dietitian or healthcare practitioner to confirm that these solutions meet your individual dietary requirements. By selecting these kidney-friendly options, you may enjoy tasty snacks and appetizers while also benefiting your kidney health.

3.5 Desserts and Sweet Treats.

Satisfying a sweet appetite while eating a healthy diet is an art.

Here's a handpicked list of desserts and sweet treats that provide the ideal balance of enjoyment.

1. **Dark chocolate-dipped strawberries**.

A traditional dessert made with antioxidant-rich dark chocolate and vitamin C-packed strawberries. The fruit's inherent sweetness balances the little bitterness of high-quality dark chocolate, resulting in a sophisticated yet easy treat.

2. **Greek yogurt parfait**

Layers of creamy Greek yogurt, mixed berries, and homemade granola make for a visually stunning dessert that's also tasty. The protein in the yogurt, along with the fiber from the fruit and granola, make this a filling and healthy meal.

3. **Baked cinnamon apples**

Core and slice apples, sprinkle with cinnamon and honey, and bake until soft. This warm, comforting dish mimics the flavor of apple pie but contains substantially fewer sugar and calories.

4. <u>**Chia seed pudding**</u>.

Chia seeds steeped in almond milk and sweetened with vanilla and a dash of maple syrup provide a creamy, pudding-like texture. Top with fresh fruit for extra natural sweetness and nutrition.

5. <u>**Frozen banana "Ice Cream"**</u>

To make dairy-free ice cream, blend frozen bananas until creamy. Add cocoa powder for a chocolate version, or a spoonful of nut butter for a richer flavor. The natural sweetness of ripe bananas eliminates the need for additional sugars.

6. <u>**Oatmeal Raisin Cookies**</u>.

These cookies, made with whole grain oats, raisins, and minimal added sugar, are high in fiber and naturally sweet. To make a lighter version, replace some of the fat with applesauce.

7. <u>**Fruit Sorbet**</u>

Blend frozen fruit with lemon juice to make a refreshing, naturally sweet sorbet. This dessert pairs particularly well with mangoes or berries.

8. **Avocado Chocolate Mousse**.

When avocado, cocoa powder, honey, and vanilla are combined, the creamy texture creates a rich mousse. It's a nutrient-dense yet surprisingly decadent treat.

9. **Poached pears**.

Poach pears in spiced tea or wine to make an attractive, low-calorie dessert. The slow cooking process enhances the fruit's natural sweetness.

10. **Frozen Yogurt Bark**

Break into pieces for a cold, refreshing treat that's strong in protein and low in added sugars.

These sweets illustrate that indulging a sweet appetite doesn't have to jeopardize your health objectives. By focusing on complete foods, natural sweetness from fruits, and attentive preparation methods, you may enjoy delectable delights that feed your body and please your palette. Moderation is crucial—even with healthier alternatives. **Savor these delicacies thoughtfully to completely enjoy their tastes and textures.**

CHAPTER 4

Lifestyle Integration and Long-Term Success.

4.1 Dining Out: Making Informed Decisions

Eating out can be difficult for people attempting to maintain a healthy diet, but with some smart planning, you can enjoy restaurant meals without jeopardizing your nutritional objectives.

Here's how to negotiate dining out and make smart, health-conscious choices:

1. **Plan ahead.**

Before going to a restaurant, look out their menu online. Many restaurants now include nutritional information, allowing you to pre-select healthier selections. This proactive strategy helps to avoid impulsive decisions motivated by hunger or temptation.

2. **Start Smart**

Start your meal with a broth-based soup or salad with dressing on the side. These low-calorie appetizers can help suppress your appetite, making you less likely to overeat higher-calorie main dishes.

3. **Decode menu language.**

Be aware of foods labeled "crispy," "breaded," "creamy," or "smothered." These words frequently suggest a greater calorie and fat content. Instead, seek for dishes marked "grilled," "steamed," "roasted," or "baked."

4. Customize your order.

Please do not hesitate to make unique requests. Request sauces and dressings on the side, vegetables instead of fries, or a meal with less oil or salt. Most establishments are willing to accommodate.

5. Practice portion control.

Restaurant servings are frequently enormous. Consider splitting a main dish, ordering an appetizer as an entree, or immediately packaging up half of your meal for later.

6. Select lean proteins.

Choose grilled fish, skinless chicken, or lean cuts of beef. These give critical nutrients without excessive saturated fat.

7. Embrace plant-based options.

Many restaurants now serve wonderful vegetarian or vegan meals. These are often lower in calories and richer in fiber and minerals.

8. Be Drink Wise

Drink water, unsweetened tea, or sparkling water with lemon. Alcoholic beverages and sugary sodas can add a lot of empty calories to your meals.

9. Slow down and savor.

Eat thoughtfully, chew gently, and savor every meal. This not only improves your meal experience, but it also allows your body to signal fullness, which prevents overeating.

10. Don't Fear Leftovers

If you are full, stop eating. There is no guilt in bringing food home. In reality, it provides an opportunity for a more balanced lunch later.

11. Educate yourself on cuisines.

Different cuisines provide healthier alternatives. For example, Mediterranean restaurants frequently provide olive oil-based meals high in healthy fats, but Japanese cuisine is known for its abundance of steaming veggies and salmon.

12. Indulge wisely.

If you decide to eat dessert, consider sharing it with your dinner guests. Alternatively, choose fruit-based desserts or a tiny amount of dark chocolate.

By using these tactics, you may achieve your nutritional objectives without giving up the enjoyment of dining out. Remember that occasional pleasures are part of a balanced existence. The idea is to make educated decisions most of the time, allowing for flexibility and enjoyment in your diet.

4.2 Adapting Family Recipes to Promote Kidney Health

One of the most typical questions I receive is,what about all of our family recipes?" It's a fair concern: food is more than simply sustenance; it's a link to our ancestors and loved ones.

The good news is that with a little imagination and know-how, you can typically modify your favorite family recipes to be kidney-friendly.

Here's how.

1. **Reduce sodium:** This is often the first step. Try halving or removing the salt in recipes.

You'd be amazed at how many meals taste better using herbs and spices rather than salt.

2. **Lower potassium:** If your kidney function is impaired, you may need to limit your potassium consumption. Replace high-potassium items with lower-potassium alternatives. For example, instead of bananas, use apples in the family fruit bread recipe.

3. **Limit phosphorus**: Many processed foods include high levels of phosphorus. In baking, use cornstarch or arrowroot powder for baking powder.

4. **Maintain protein balance**: While protein is essential, too much might stress damaged kidneys. In meat-heavy meals, consider using less meat and more veggies.

5. **Keep portion proportions in mind:** You can sometimes stick with a recipe but eat a lower quantity.

Begin with your family's favorite dishes and work on altering them one by one. It may even become a fun family project if everyone participates in taste-testing the new variations!

I usually remind my patients that this path is about achieving balance, not perfectionism. There may be occasions when you want to consume a tiny bit of the original dish as a pleasure. That is alright! The trick is to make educated decisions most of the time.

Do not be scared to start new customs. Perhaps your altered recipes will become new family favorites that future generations will treasure. Your health journey might start a new chapter in your family's culinary history.

4.3 Managing Social Situations and Special Events.

Manage social situations and special occasions:

1. **Before dining out**, research menus since many establishments now offer them online. Before you leave, look for choices that are good for your kidneys.

Communicate with the server. Do not hesitate to inquire about ingredients or preparation procedures. Most eateries are ready to meet dietary requirements.

Make sensible choices: choose grilled, baked, or steamed meals over fried items.

Portion control: Restaurants frequently provide big amounts. Consider splitting a meal or asking for a takeout box immediately.

2. **For family gatherings, bring a meal**. Contribute a kidney-friendly meal to ensure you have something to eat.

Inform your host. Make them aware of your dietary requirements ahead of time. Most hosts appreciate the notice and will attempt to accommodate.

Concentrate on socialization: Remember that parties are about more than simply food. Enjoy the company and the chat.

3. **Plan ahead:** Many holiday meals have high levels of salt, potassium, and phosphorus. Work with your dietician to develop a holiday food plan.

Modify traditions. Find new ways to prepare traditional holiday meals. For example, in baking, use unsalted butter and replace sweet potatoes with turnips.

Start new traditions: Create new holiday traditions that do not include food, such as a family game night or a volunteer activity.

4. **Tips for Parties and Celebrations**: Eat a modest, kidney-friendly meal beforehand to avoid temptation.

Make intelligent choices at the buffet. Choose fresh fruits and vegetables, lean meats, and avoid highly processed meals.

Stay hydrated: If you are on a hydration restriction, monitor your consumption. Alternate between water and other beverages if permitted.

5. **Before consuming alcohol, see your doctor.** Some renal patients may need to avoid alcohol totally, but others may be able to use it in moderation.

Be wary of the hidden phosphorus: Beer and dark colas are very rich in phosphorus.

Stay hydrated: If you drink, be sure to consume water in between alcoholic beverages.

6. **Travel: Plan meals**. Research eateries on your trip. Consider arranging rooms that have a kitchen so you may make your own meals.

Pack food: Bring kidney-friendly snacks for the trip and to have on hand at your destination.

Medication management: Make sure you have adequate medication for your journey, with extra in case of delays.

7. **Workplace Situations**: Educate coworkers: If possible, notify close colleagues about your dietary requirements to prevent unpleasant situations.

Be prepared. Keep kidney-friendly snacks on your desk for unexpected workplace treats or lunches.

Navigate Business Meals: When feasible, recommend eateries where you know you'll find appropriate selections.

8. Emotional Aspects: Acknowledge feelings: It's acceptable to feel irritated or excluded at times. These sentiments are real and widespread among renal sufferers.

Seek help: Think about joining a renal patient support group. Sharing experiences may be really beneficial.

Concentrate on what you can eat: Rather than obsessing on restricted meals, appreciate the numerous tasty alternatives that are still available to you.

9. **Communicating with loved ones**: Be open. Explain your dietary requirements to your

close friends and family. Most people want to be helpful, but they may not understand unless explained.

___Provide alternatives:__ If someone wants to treat you to a dinner, choose a kidney-friendly restaurant or a non-food activity instead.

10. **Maintaining Perspective:** Focus on your overall health. One off-plan meal will not destroy your progress, but frequent decisions do.

_______Celebrate non-food victories:__ Use changes in your test results, energy levels, or overall well-being as motivation to stay to your strategy.

Maintaining kidney health is a journey, not a destination. There may be difficulties, but with preparation and the appropriate mentality, you can handle social settings and special occasions while still living life to the fullest. The objective is to strike a balance that allows you to attend social events, retain cultural and family traditions, and care for your health.

4.4 Tracking Progress: Monitoring Diet and Kidney Function

Monitoring both your diet and kidney function provides crucial information about how well your treatment strategy is working.

Let us break this down into actual, actionable measures.

1. **Diet Tracking:**
   1. a) Food Diary: Keep a complete diary of your eating and drinking habits for at least one week every month.

Take note of the quantity proportions, cooking techniques, and any seasonings used.

There are several applications available for this, or you simply keep a simple notepad.

   1. b) Nutrient Analysis: Collaborate with a renal dietitian to assess your food diary.

Concentrate on essential nutrients such as salt, potassium, phosphorus, and protein.

Try to find trends and opportunities for improvement.

1. c) **Fluid consumption:** If on fluid restrictions, carefully monitor your daily consumption.

Remember that items like soup, jello, and ice cream count as fluid consumption.

2. **Monitor Kidney Function:**

2.a) Regular Blood Tests: We typically examine your blood every 3-6 months, or more frequently as needed.

The key markers we look at are:

Blood Urea Nitrogen (BUN): measures kidney function * Electrolytes: potassium, sodium, and phosphorus * Hemoglobin: detects anemia, which is frequent with renal disease

2.b) Urine Tests: We may do frequent urinalysis to detect protein or blood in your urine.

A 24-hour urine sample can provide more specific information about your kidney function and how effectively your body handles different chemicals.

2.c) Blood Pressure Monitoring: High blood pressure can both cause and worsen renal disease.

Aim for the objective we outlined, which is often less than 130/80 for most renal patients.

3. **Body Composition**

3.a) Weight: Weigh yourself frequently, preferably at the same time every day.

Sudden weight increase may suggest fluid retention.

3.b) Edema: Check for swelling, especially in ankles and feet. Please let us know if you notice any additional puffiness or if your shoes feel tighter.

4. **Symptom tracking:**

Keep a record of any symptoms you notice, such as weariness, nausea, urine changes, or muscular cramping.

Take note of when symptoms appear and any possible triggers.

5. **Medication adherence:**

Use a pill organizer or app to ensure that you are taking all of your recommended prescriptions.

Keep track of any adverse effects and discuss them with your healthcare staff.

6. **Regular Check-Ups:**

Keep all planned visits with your renal care team.

Bring your tracking records along with any questions you may have.

7. **Technology Aids:**

Consider utilizing kidney-specific applications to track all these aspects in one spot. Some apps can even deliver reports straight to your healthcare staff.

8. **Collaborative approach:**

Share your tracking data with your renal care team, including your nephrologist, primary care doctor, dietician, and other experts. This allows us to make educated judgments regarding your treatment strategy.

9. **Setting goals:**

Collaborate with your care team to create realistic, attainable goals.

Celebrate when you achieve these goals, no matter how tiny they may appear.

10. <u>Adjusting Your Plan:</u>

Depending on your monitoring data and test findings, we may need to change your diet, medicines, or other components of your treatment plan.

This is a dynamic process; what works today may need to be tweaked tomorrow.

Remember that measuring your progress is not about perfection. It is about obtaining information to help us make the best health decisions for you. Some days will be better than others, and that's fine. The aim is to show an overall improvement over time.

By routinely monitoring your diet and renal function, we can detect problems early and make appropriate changes. This preventative strategy can decrease the course of kidney disease and make you feel better.

CONCLUSION

Sarah Thompson's life fell when she heard the words **"stage 3 chronic kidney disease" at the age of 32.** A vivacious chef with a thriving catering business, she suddenly found herself facing a future in which her enthusiasm for food appeared to conflict with her health. The kitchen, once her haven, had become a labyrinth of banned items and perplexing constraints.

This cookbook chronicles Sarah's journey from despair to optimism, from feeling betrayed by her own body to rediscovering her love of cooking and eating. With frank honesty, she relates her tears over favorite recipes that are suddenly off-limits, her irritation with bland hospital meals, and the moment she nearly gave up on her life's purpose.

But **Sarah's** story does not end there. It demonstrates human perseverance and innovation. Sarah created a fresh approach to cooking via trial and error, many interactions with other patients and renal dietitians, and a steadfast commitment to live rather than merely survive.

These sections include more than simply kidney-friendly recipes. They are imbued with Sarah's contagious positivity and hard-earned knowledge. From replicating her grandmother's favorite lasagna to creating holiday feasts that don't jeopardize her health, each dish is a celebration of life and a challenge to restrictions.

Sarah's exploits (such as the Great Salt-Free Bread Disaster of 2018) will make you laugh, weep, and celebrate. Most significantly, you'll get a companion and advisor throughout your renal health journey.

This is not only a cookbook. **It's a lifeline for everyone who has ever felt overwhelmed by dietary constraints.** It demonstrates that a diagnosis does not define you and that with the correct tools and approach, you can not only nourish your kidneys but also regain the joy of eating and life.

Whether you're recently diagnosed, a seasoned fighter, or cooking for a loved one with kidney disease, Sarah's narrative and recipes will motivate you to take control of your health without compromising flavor or pleasure. Prepare to convert your kitchen into a haven of healing, hope, and culinary possibilities.